Table of Contents

INTRODUCTION

I welcome you to the world of healthy and delicious eating! If you're seeking a culinary adventure that combines the benefits of a low-sodium diet with the goodness of plant-based ingredients, you're in the right place. This Low Sodium Plant-Based Cookbook is your passport to a flavorful, heart-healthy lifestyle that doesn't compromise on taste or nutrition.

In today's fast-paced world, many of us are becoming increasingly aware of the importance of our dietary choices. High sodium intake has been linked to various health issues, including hypertension and heart disease. But that doesn't mean you have to give up on taste and satisfaction. With this cookbook, we aim to show you that reducing your sodium intake doesn't mean sacrificing flavor or variety.

What to Expect in this Cookbook:

• Delicious and Nutrient-Rich Recipes: My cookbook is filled with mouthwatering recipes that highlight the natural flavors of plant-based ingredients. From vibrant salads and hearty soups to satisfying main courses and delectable desserts, you'll find a wide range of options to tantalize your taste buds.

• Low Sodium Guidelines: I provide guidance on reducing sodium in your diet without compromising on taste. I'll teach you how to use herbs, spices, and other flavor-enhancing techniques to create dishes that are both heart-healthy and delicious.

• Nutritional Information: Each recipe comes with detailed nutritional information, including sodium content, so you can make informed choices about your meals.

• Cooking Tips and Tricks: Whether you're a seasoned chef or a beginner in the kitchen, my cookbook offers valuable tips and techniques to make your plant-based, low sodium cooking experience enjoyable and effortless.

• Diverse and Inclusive: I celebrate the diversity of plant-based eating by including recipes inspired by various cuisines from around the world. There's something for everyone, regardless of your dietary preferences or restrictions.

• Health Benefits: Throughout the cookbook, I'll share insights into the health benefits of the ingredients used in each recipe, so you can better understand how your choices are positively impacting your well-being.

• This Low Sodium Plant-Based Cookbook is not just a collection of recipes; it's a lifestyle guide that empowers you to take control of your health and savor the joys of flavorful, plant-based eating. I invite you to explore these pages, experiment in your kitchen, and embark on a culinary journey that promises not only delectable meals but also a healthier and happier you.

So, grab your apron, sharpen your knives, and let's embark on this delicious and healthful adventure together! Your heart and taste buds will thank you.

WHY CHOOSE A LOW SODIUM, PLANT-BASED DIET?

Plant-based diets have gained immense popularity in recent years for their numerous health benefits. They are rich in vitamins, minerals, fiber, and antioxidants, while being low in saturated fats and cholesterol. Such diets have been shown to reduce the risk of chronic diseases, improve weight management, and promote overall well-being.

Additionally, a low sodium diet can help lower blood pressure, reduce the risk of stroke, and protect your heart. By combining the principles of a plant-based diet with low sodium guidelines, you're embarking on a journey toward better health and vitality.

Low sodium guidelines are essential for individuals who want to reduce their sodium intake for health reasons, such as managing high blood pressure, preventing heart disease, or improving overall well-being. Here are some key guidelines to follow when adopting a low sodium diet:

• Know Your Daily Limit: It's important to understand the recommended daily limit for sodium intake. In general, the Dietary Guidelines for Americans recommend consuming less than 2,300 milligrams (mg) of sodium per day, which is about one teaspoon of salt. However, for specific populations, such as adults over 50, African Americans, and those with certain health conditions, the recommended limit is even lower, at 1,500 mg per day.

• Read Food Labels: One of the most effective ways to control your sodium intake is by reading food labels carefully. Pay attention to the "Sodium" content listed on packaged foods. Choose products labeled as "low sodium" or "no added salt" whenever possible.

• Cook at Home: Preparing meals at home allows you to have greater control over the sodium content of your food. When cooking, use fresh ingredients and limit the use of processed and pre-packaged foods, which often contain high levels of sodium.

• Use Herbs and Spices: Instead of relying on salt for flavor, experiment with a variety of herbs, spices, and seasonings to enhance the taste of your dishes. Some options include garlic, basil, oregano, rosemary, lemon juice, vinegar, and low-sodium seasoning blends.

• Limit Salt in Cooking: When cooking, use less salt than a recipe suggests or omit it entirely. You can always add a small amount at the end if needed, but you may find that your taste buds adapt to lower sodium levels over time.

• Choose Fresh Produce: Fruits and vegetables are naturally low in sodium and high in essential nutrients. Incorporate a wide variety of fresh produce into your diet to boost flavor and nutrition.

• Select Low-Sodium or No-Salt-Added Products: When purchasing canned or processed foods, look for options labeled as "low sodium" or "no salt added." These products often have significantly less sodium than their regular counterparts.

• Be Cautious with Condiments and Sauces: Condiments like soy sauce, ketchup, and salad dressings can be high in sodium. Opt for low-sodium or reduced-sodium versions, or consider making your own sauces and dressings at home.

• Limit Processed Meats: Processed meats like bacon, ham, sausages, and deli meats are typically high in sodium. Choose lean cuts of fresh meat, poultry, or seafood, and prepare them without adding excessive salt.

• Monitor Restaurant Choices: When dining out,
ask for dishes to be prepared with less salt or sauce
on the side. Many restaurants now offer low-
sodium menu options or can accommodate special
dietary requests.

• Stay Hydrated: Drinking plenty of water can help
flush excess sodium from your body. Aim for at
least eight 8-ounce glasses of water per day, and
consider reducing your intake of high-sodium
beverages like soda.

• Plan Balanced Meals: Focus on creating balanced
meals that include a variety of foods from different
food groups. This helps ensure you get the
nutrients you need while managing your sodium
intake.

NUTRITIONAL INFORMATION

Nutritional information is a key component of
understanding the content of the food you eat and
making informed dietary choices. It provides details

about the composition of a food item, including its macronutrients (carbohydrates, proteins, and fats), micronutrients (vitamins and minerals), and other relevant factors like calories and serving size. Here's an overview of the important elements typically included in nutritional information:

Serving Size: This indicates the amount of the food product that the provided nutritional information applies to. It's important to pay attention to serving size because the nutrient content is based on this portion.

Calories: The number of calories in a serving of the food is listed. Calories provide energy for the body, and understanding their content can help with managing your daily energy intake.

Macronutrients:

Carbohydrates: This includes total carbohydrates and may break down further into dietary fiber and sugars. Carbohydrates are a primary source of energy.

Proteins: The amount of protein per serving is typically listed. Protein is essential for growth, repair, and various bodily functions.

Fats: The total fat content is provided, with a breakdown of saturated and trans fats, which are less healthy, and unsaturated fats, which are generally considered healthier.

Micronutrients:

Vitamins: Nutritional information often includes information about the presence and quantity of vitamins, such as vitamin A, vitamin C, calcium, and iron.

Minerals: Information about minerals like sodium, potassium, magnesium, and others may be included.

Percent Daily Value (DV): This percentage tells you how much a nutrient in a serving of the food contributes to your daily recommended intake. It's based on a daily diet of 2,000 calories, which may vary depending on your individual needs. For example, if a food item has 15% DV of calcium, it means it provides 15% of the recommended daily intake for calcium based on a 2,000-calorie diet.

Ingredients List: Some food labels include an ingredients list, which shows the components used to make the product. Ingredients are typically listed in descending order by weight, with the most prominent ingredient listed first.

Allergen Information: If a product contains common allergens like nuts, dairy, wheat, or soy, it should be clearly indicated in the ingredients list or a separate allergen statement.

Additional Nutrient Information: Depending on the product, additional information may be provided, such as cholesterol, dietary fiber, sugars, and others.

Nutrient Claims: Some foods may include specific nutrient claims, such as "low in fat," "high in fiber," or "excellent source of vitamin C," to highlight certain nutritional characteristics.

Reading and understanding nutritional information can help you make healthier food choices, track your nutrient intake, and manage specific dietary needs or restrictions. When using this information, consider your individual nutritional requirements, dietary goals, and any health conditions you may have to make informed decisions about the foods you consume.

COOKING TIPS AND TRICKS

Cooking is not just a skill; it's an art. Whether you're a beginner or an experienced cook, there are always tips and tricks to enhance your culinary prowess. Here are some valuable cooking tips and tricks to make your time in the kitchen more enjoyable and successful:

1. Read the Recipe First:

Before you start cooking, thoroughly read the recipe to understand the steps, ingredients, and equipment needed. This prevents surprises and helps you plan better.

2. Prep Ingredients in Advance:

Mise en place, a French term meaning "everything in its place," is a fundamental concept. Prepare and measure all your ingredients before you start cooking. This saves time and reduces stress during cooking.

3. Invest in Quality Tools:

Good quality knives, cookware, and utensils can make a significant difference in your cooking experience. Invest in the essentials for your kitchen.

4. Keep Your Workspace Organized:

Maintain a clean and organized cooking area. This not only makes cooking more efficient but also safer.

5. Taste as You Go:

Taste your food throughout the cooking process to adjust seasoning and flavors as needed. This prevents over-salting or under-seasoning dishes.

6. Use Fresh Ingredients:

Whenever possible, use fresh and seasonal ingredients for the best flavor and nutrition. Fresh herbs, spices, and produce can elevate your dishes.

7. Control Your Heat:

Learn how to control the heat on your stovetop. Different dishes require different heat levels, from low simmering to high searing.

8. Don't Crowd the Pan:

When sautéing or frying, avoid overcrowding the pan, as it can lead to uneven cooking and steaming rather than browning.

9. Master Basic Techniques:

Focus on mastering fundamental cooking techniques like chopping, sautéing, roasting, and braising. These skills form the foundation for a wide range of dishes.

10. Experiment with Flavors:

- Be adventurous with herbs, spices, and seasonings to create unique flavor profiles. Mix and match ingredients to discover your own culinary style.

11. Embrace Resting Time:

- Let cooked meats rest before slicing. Resting allows the juices to redistribute, resulting in juicier, more flavorful cuts.

12. Use a Timer:

- Timers are your best friends in the kitchen. They help you avoid overcooking or burning dishes.

13. Keep Stock and Basic Ingredients On Hand:

- Maintain a well-stocked pantry with essentials like olive oil, vinegar, flour, sugar, canned tomatoes, and broth. This ensures you can whip up a meal even on short notice.

14. Learn Knife Skills:

- Proper knife skills not only improve safety but also make food prep faster and more enjoyable.

15. Taste with Your Senses:

- Pay attention to the aroma, texture, and appearance of your dishes. Cooking is as much about senses as it is about taste.

16. Be Patient: -

Some dishes require time and patience. Slow-cooked stews, for example, develop deep flavors over time.

17. Don't Be Afraid to Fail:

- Mistakes happen to everyone. Learn from them and use them as opportunities for growth in your culinary journey.

18. Document Your Creations:

- Keep a cooking journal to record your successful recipes and experiments. This helps you replicate your favorite dishes and track your culinary progress.

HEALTH BENEFITS

Adopting a plant-based diet that's low in sodium offers a wide range of health benefits. Here are some of the significant advantages of following a low sodium, plant-based diet:

Heart Health: Reduced sodium intake can help lower blood pressure, reducing the risk of hypertension and heart disease. Plant-based diets are also naturally low in saturated fats and cholesterol, further promoting heart health.

Lowered Stroke Risk: By controlling blood pressure, a low sodium diet decreases the risk of strokes, which are often linked to high blood pressure.

Weight Management: Plant-based diets tend to be lower in calories and saturated fats, making them effective for weight management and obesity prevention.

Improved Digestion: A diet rich in plant-based foods, such as fruits, vegetables, and whole grains, provides dietary fiber that aids in digestion and can help prevent constipation.

Reduced Cancer Risk: Some studies suggest that plant-based diets may reduce the risk of certain cancers, including colon, breast, and prostate cancers.

Better Blood Sugar Control: Plant-based diets can help stabilize blood sugar levels, making them beneficial for individuals with diabetes or those at risk of developing diabetes.

Kidney Health: Lower sodium intake is essential for individuals with kidney issues, as it reduces the workload on the kidneys and helps manage conditions like chronic kidney disease.

Bone Health: A plant-based diet can be rich in calcium, which is essential for bone health. Foods like leafy greens, almonds, and fortified plant-based milk can contribute to strong bones.

Reduced Inflammation: Plant-based diets are often associated with lower levels of inflammation in the body, which can help prevent chronic inflammatory conditions.

Improved Digestive Health: The fiber in plant-based foods supports a healthy gut microbiome, promoting good digestive health and reducing the risk of gastrointestinal issues.

Longevity: Studies have shown that plant-based diets are associated with a longer lifespan and a reduced risk of premature death from various causes.

Improved Skin Health: A diet rich in fruits and vegetables provides vitamins and antioxidants that promote healthy skin and may reduce the signs of aging.

Environmental Benefits: Plant-based diets have a lower environmental impact compared to diets high in animal products. Reducing meat and dairy consumption can contribute to a more sustainable planet.

Ethical Considerations: Many people choose plant-based diets for ethical reasons, as they involve less harm to animals and promote more humane and sustainable agricultural practices.

Mental Well-Being: Some individuals report improved mood and mental clarity when following a plant-based diet, which may be attributed to the

nutrients found in plant-based foods.

LOW SODIUM PLANT BASED COOKBOOK

Veggie Stir-Fry

• Ingredients:

• Mixed vegetables (e.g., bell peppers, broccoli, carrots, snap peas)

• Low-sodium soy sauce or tamari

• Garlic and ginger (minced)

• Tofu or tempeh (cubed)

• Sesame oil

Instructions:

• Heat sesame oil in a pan and sauté garlic and ginger.

• Add tofu or tempeh and cook until lightly browned.

• Add vegetables and stir-fry until tender.

• Finish with a splash of low-sodium soy sauce.

Lentil and Vegetable Curry

Ingredients:

• Red lentils

• Mixed vegetables (e.g., cauliflower, spinach, carrots)

• Curry paste or powder

• Coconut milk (low-sodium)

• Onion and garlic (chopped)

Instructions:

• Sauté onion and garlic in a pot.

• Add curry paste/powder and cook briefly.

• Add lentils, vegetables, and coconut milk.

• Simmer until lentils are tender.

Chickpea and Spinach Stew

Ingredients:

• Chickpeas (canned or cooked)

• Spinach

• Tomatoes (canned or fresh)

• Onion and garlic (chopped)

• Cumin and coriander (ground)

Instructions:

• Sauté onion and garlic in a large pot.

• Add cumin and coriander and cook briefly.

• Add chickpeas, tomatoes, and spinach.

• Simmer until spinach wilts.

Mushroom and Spinach Quinoa

Ingredients:

• Quinoa

- Mushrooms (sliced)

- Spinach

- Vegetable broth (low-sodium)

- Onion and garlic (chopped)

Instructions:

- Sauté onion and garlic in a pan.

- Add mushrooms and cook until tender.

- Stir in quinoa and vegetable broth.

- Simmer until quinoa is cooked.

- Mix in spinach until wilted.

Stuffed Bell Peppers

Ingredients:

- Bell peppers

- Brown rice

- Black beans (canned)

• Corn kernels

• Tomato sauce (low-sodium)

Instructions:

• Cook brown rice and mix with beans and corn.

• Stuff bell peppers with the rice mixture.

• Place stuffed peppers in a baking dish, pour tomato sauce over them, and bake until peppers are tender.

Spaghetti Squash with Marinara

Ingredients:

• Spaghetti squash

• Tomatoes (canned or fresh)

• Onion and garlic (chopped)

• Basil and oregano (dried)

Instructions:

- Roast or microwave spaghetti squash until tender.

- Sauté onion and garlic, then add tomatoes and spices for marinara sauce.

- Scrape squash into strands and serve with sauce.

Vegan Chili

Ingredients:

- Kidney beans (canned)

- Black beans (canned)

- Diced tomatoes (canned)

- Chili powder and cumin (ground)

- Onion and garlic (chopped)

Instructions:

- Sauté onion and garlic, then add beans, tomatoes, and spices.

• Simmer until flavors meld.

Vegan Shepherd's Pie

Ingredients:

• Lentils (cooked)

• Mixed vegetables (e.g., peas, carrots)

• Mashed potatoes (made with low-sodium vegetable broth)

Instructions:

• Layer cooked lentils and vegetables in a baking dish.

• Top with mashed potatoes.

• Bake until the top is golden brown.

Mushroom and Spinach Vegan Lasagna

Ingredients:

- Whole wheat lasagna noodles

- Mushrooms (sliced)

- Spinach

- Vegan ricotta cheese

- Tomato sauce (low-sodium)

Instructions:

- Layer noodles with mushrooms, spinach, vegan ricotta, and tomato sauce.

- Bake until bubbly.

Black Bean and Sweet Potato Tacos

Ingredients:

- Black beans (canned)

- Sweet potatoes (roasted and mashed)

- Taco shells (whole wheat)

- Salsa (low-sodium)

Instructions:

• Fill taco shells with mashed sweet potatoes, black beans, and salsa.

Veggie and Tofu Stir-Fry

Ingredients:

• Mixed vegetables (e.g., bell peppers, broccoli, snap peas)

• Tofu (cubed)

• Low-sodium teriyaki sauce

• Garlic and ginger (minced)

Instructions:

• Sauté garlic and ginger, add tofu, and cook until browned.

• Add vegetables and stir-fry with teriyaki sauce.

Quinoa and Chickpea Salad

Ingredients:

• Quinoa

• Chickpeas (canned)

• Cucumber, tomatoes, and red onion (chopped)

• Lemon juice and olive oil (dressing)

Instructions:

• Cook quinoa and mix with chickpeas and vegetables.

• Drizzle with lemon juice and olive oil.

Vegan Lentil Soup

Ingredients:

• Red lentils

• Carrots, celery, and onions (chopped)

• Vegetable broth (low-sodium)

• Cumin and turmeric (ground)

Instructions:

• Sauté vegetables, add lentils, broth, and spices.

• Simmer until lentils are soft.

Tofu and Vegetable Curry

Ingredients:

• Tofu (cubed)

• Mixed vegetables (e.g., bell peppers, peas, carrots)

• Curry paste or powder

• Coconut milk (low-sodium)

Instructions:

• Sauté tofu and vegetables, then add curry paste and coconut milk.

• Simmer until heated through.

Vegan Mediterranean Bowl

Ingredients:

• Quinoa or brown rice

• Chickpeas (canned)

• Cucumber, tomatoes, olives, and red onion (chopped)

• Tahini dressing

Instructions:

• Layer cooked quinoa or rice with chickpeas, vegetables, and tahini dressing.

Vegan Broccoli and Cashew Stir-Fry

Ingredients:

• Broccoli florets

• Cashews

• Bell peppers (sliced)

• Low-sodium stir-fry sauce

Instructions:

• Stir-fry broccoli, cashews, and bell peppers with
stir-fry sauce.

Vegan Eggplant Parmesan

Ingredients:

• Eggplant slices (breaded and baked)

• Vegan marinara sauce (low-sodium)

• Vegan mozzarella cheese

Instructions:

• Layer eggplant slices with marinara sauce and
vegan cheese, then bake until bubbly.

Vegan Thai Green Curry

Ingredients:

• Mixed vegetables (e.g., bell peppers, zucchini, snow peas)

• Tofu or tempeh (cubed)

• Thai green curry paste

• Coconut milk (low-sodium)

Instructions:

• Sauté tofu or tempeh, add vegetables, curry paste, and coconut milk.

• Simmer until heated through.

Vegan Mediterranean Stuffed Bell Peppers

Ingredients:

• Bell peppers

• Quinoa

• Chickpeas (canned)

- Diced tomatoes (canned)

- Olive tapenade

Instructions:

- Cook quinoa and mix with chickpeas, diced tomatoes, and olive tapenade.

- Stuff bell peppers and bake until tender.

Vegan Lentil Loaf

Ingredients:

- Green lentils (cooked)

- Oats

- Carrots, celery, and onions (chopped)

- Vegan tomato-based sauce (low-sodium)

Instructions:

- Mix cooked lentils, oats, vegetables, and tomato sauce.

• Form into a loaf shape and bake until firm.

Quinoa and Black Bean Salad

Ingredients:

• Cooked quinoa

• Black beans (canned)

• Corn kernels (fresh or frozen)

• Red bell pepper (chopped)

• Lime juice and cilantro (for dressing)

Instructions:

• Mix cooked quinoa, black beans, corn, and red bell pepper.

• Drizzle with a dressing made from lime juice and chopped cilantro.

Roasted Garlic and Herb Vegetables

Ingredients:

• Assorted vegetables (e.g., carrots, potatoes, zucchini)

• Garlic (whole cloves)

• Fresh herbs (e.g., rosemary, thyme)

• Olive oil (low-sodium)

Instructions:

• Toss vegetables, garlic cloves, and herbs with olive oil.

• Roast in the oven until tender and lightly browned.

Cauliflower Mashed Potatoes

Ingredients:

• Cauliflower florets

• Potatoes (peeled and diced)

• Nutritional yeast (for flavor)

• Garlic (minced)

Instructions:

• Steam cauliflower and potatoes until soft.

• Mash together with nutritional yeast and minced garlic.

Vegan Coleslaw

Ingredients:

• Shredded cabbage and carrots

• Vegan mayo

• Dijon mustard

• Apple cider vinegar

• Celery seeds (optional)

Instructions:

• Mix shredded cabbage and carrots with a dressing made from vegan mayo, Dijon mustard, apple cider vinegar, and celery seeds.

Garlic Lemon Roasted Asparagus

Ingredients:

• Asparagus spears

• Garlic (minced)

• Lemon juice and zest

• Olive oil (low-sodium)

Instructions:

• Toss asparagus with minced garlic, lemon juice, lemon zest, and a drizzle of olive oil.

• Roast until tender.

Balsamic Glazed Brussels Sprouts

Ingredients:

• Brussels sprouts (halved)

• Balsamic vinegar

• Maple syrup

Instructions:

• Roast Brussels sprouts until crisp-tender.

• Toss with a glaze made from balsamic vinegar and maple syrup.

Vegan Greek Salad

Ingredients:

• Cucumber, tomatoes, red onion, and Kalamata olives (chopped)

• Vegan feta cheese

• Fresh oregano (chopped)

• Lemon juice and olive oil (low-sodium)

Instructions:

• Combine chopped vegetables, vegan feta, and oregano.

• Drizzle with a dressing made from lemon juice and olive oil.

Herbed Quinoa

Ingredients:

• Cooked quinoa

• Fresh herbs (e.g., parsley, mint, dill)

• Lemon juice and olive oil (low-sodium)

Instructions:

• Mix cooked quinoa with chopped fresh herbs.

• Drizzle with a dressing made from lemon juice and olive oil.

Vegan Creamed Spinach

Ingredients:

• Fresh spinach

• Cashew cream (blended cashews and water)

• Nutmeg (for flavor)

Instructions:

• Sauté fresh spinach until wilted.

• Stir in cashew cream and a pinch of nutmeg.

Mango Salsa

Ingredients:

• Mango (diced)

• Red onion (finely chopped)

• Fresh cilantro (chopped)

• Lime juice

Instructions:

- Mix diced mango, chopped red onion, chopped cilantro, and lime juice.

Cauliflower Rice

Ingredients:

- Cauliflower florets (riced in a food processor)

- Garlic (minced)

- Turmeric (for color and flavor)

Instructions:

- Sauté riced cauliflower with minced garlic and a pinch of turmeric until tender.

Lemon Dill Cucumber Salad

Ingredients:

- Cucumbers (sliced)

- Fresh dill (chopped)

• Lemon juice and olive oil (low-sodium)

Instructions:

• Combine sliced cucumbers and chopped fresh dill.

• Drizzle with a dressing made from lemon juice and olive oil.

Roasted Sweet Potato Wedges

Ingredients:

• Sweet potatoes (cut into wedges)

• Paprika and cayenne pepper (for seasoning)

• Olive oil (low-sodium)

Instructions:

• Toss sweet potato wedges with paprika, cayenne pepper, and a drizzle of olive oil.

• Roast until crisp and golden.

Vegan Tabbouleh

Ingredients:

• Bulgur wheat (cooked)

• Fresh parsley, mint, and tomatoes (chopped)

• Lemon juice and olive oil (low-sodium)

Instructions:

• Mix cooked bulgur with chopped fresh herbs, tomatoes, and a dressing made from lemon juice and olive oil.

Sesame Cucumber Noodles

Ingredients:

• Cucumbers (spiraled into noodles)

• Sesame seeds

• Rice vinegar and sesame oil (low-sodium)

Instructions:

• Toss cucumber noodles with sesame seeds and a dressing made from rice vinegar and sesame oil.

Vegan Stuffed Mushrooms

Ingredients:

• Large mushrooms (stems removed)

• Spinach and garlic (sautéed)

• Vegan bread crumbs

Instructions:

• Stuff mushrooms with sautéed spinach and garlic, then top with vegan bread crumbs.

• Bake until mushrooms are tender.

Vegan Ratatouille

Ingredients:

• Eggplant, zucchini, bell peppers, and tomatoes (sliced)

• Garlic and basil (minced)

• Olive oil (low-sodium)

Instructions:

• Layer sliced vegetables with minced garlic and basil.

• Drizzle with a little olive oil and bake until tender.

Vegan Caprese Salad

Ingredients:

• Tomatoes and fresh basil leaves

• Vegan mozzarella cheese

• Balsamic glaze

Instructions:

• Layer tomato slices, basil leaves, and slices of vegan mozzarella.

• Drizzle with balsamic glaze.

Vegan Cabbage Slaw

Ingredients:

• Shredded green and purple cabbage

• Vegan mayo

• Apple cider vinegar and Dijon mustard

• Celery seeds (optional)

Instructions:

• Mix shredded cabbage with a dressing made from vegan mayo, apple cider vinegar, Dijon mustard, and celery seeds.

Vegan Garlic Roasted Broccoli

Ingredients:

• Broccoli florets

• Garlic (minced)

• Olive oil (low-sodium)

Instructions:

• Toss broccoli with minced garlic and a drizzle of olive oil.

• Roast until tender and lightly browned.

SOUP

Lentil Soup

Ingredients:

• Red lentils

• Carrots, celery, and onions (chopped)

• Vegetable broth (low-sodium)

• Cumin and turmeric (ground)

Instructions:

• Sauté vegetables, add lentils, broth, and spices.

• Simmer until lentils are soft.

Vegan Minestrone

Ingredients:

• Cannellini beans (canned)

• Tomatoes (canned or fresh)

• Mixed vegetables (e.g., zucchini, spinach)

• Whole wheat pasta

Instructions:

• Combine beans, tomatoes, and vegetables in a pot.

• Add whole wheat pasta and simmer until cooked.

Butternut Squash Soup

Ingredients:

• Butternut squash (cubed)

• Onion and garlic (chopped)

• Vegetable broth (low-sodium)

• Nutmeg (for flavor)

Instructions:

• Sauté onion and garlic, add squash and broth, and simmer until tender.

• Purée and season with nutmeg.

Vegan Potato Leek Soup

Ingredients:

• Potatoes (peeled and diced)

• Leeks (sliced)

• Vegetable broth (low-sodium)

• Cashew cream (blended cashews and water)

Instructions:

• Sauté leeks, add potatoes and broth, and simmer until potatoes are soft.

• Stir in cashew cream.

Tomato Basil Soup

Ingredients:

• Tomatoes (canned or fresh)

• Fresh basil (chopped)

• Onion and garlic (chopped)

• Olive oil (low-sodium)

Instructions:

• Sauté onion and garlic, add tomatoes and basil, and simmer.

• Purée and season with olive oil.

Vegan Broccoli Soup

Ingredients:

• Broccoli florets

• Onion and garlic (chopped)

• Vegetable broth (low-sodium)

• Nutritional yeast (for flavor)

Instructions:

• Sauté onion and garlic, add broccoli and broth, and simmer until tender.

• Purée and stir in nutritional yeast.

Vegan Spinach and Artichoke Soup

Ingredients:

• Fresh spinach

• Canned artichoke hearts

• Onion and garlic (chopped)

• Vegetable broth (low-sodium)

Instructions:

• Sauté onion and garlic, add spinach, artichoke hearts, and broth.

• Simmer until spinach wilts.

Vegan Carrot Ginger Soup

Ingredients:

• Carrots (sliced)

• Ginger (minced)

• Vegetable broth (low-sodium)

• Coconut milk (low-sodium)

Instructions:

• Sauté carrots and ginger, add broth, and simmer until carrots are tender.

• Purée and stir in coconut milk.

Vegan Cauliflower Soup

Ingredients:

• Cauliflower florets

• Onion and garlic (chopped)

• Vegetable broth (low-sodium)

• Dijon mustard (for flavor)

Instructions:

• Sauté onion and garlic, add cauliflower and broth, and simmer until tender.

• Purée and season with Dijon mustard.

Vegan Asparagus Soup

Ingredients:

• Asparagus spears

• Onion and garlic (chopped)

• Vegetable broth (low-sodium)

• Lemon juice and zest

Instructions:

• Sauté onion and garlic, add asparagus, broth, and simmer until asparagus is tender.

• Purée and season with lemon juice and zest.

Vegan Mushroom Soup

Ingredients:

• Mushrooms (sliced)

• Onion and garlic (chopped)

• Vegetable broth (low-sodium)

• Thyme and rosemary (dried)

Instructions:

• Sauté mushrooms, onion, and garlic until browned.

- Add broth and dried herbs, and simmer.

- Purée and season with salt-free seasonings.

Vegan Split Pea Soup

Ingredients:

- Green split peas

- Carrots, celery, and onions (chopped)

- Vegetable broth (low-sodium)

- Bay leaves (for flavor)

Instructions:

- Combine split peas, vegetables, broth, and bay leaves in a pot.

- Simmer until peas are soft.

Vegan Sweet Potato Soup

Ingredients:

• Sweet potatoes (peeled and diced)

• Onion and garlic (chopped)

• Vegetable broth (low-sodium)

• Coconut milk (low-sodium)

Instructions:

• Sauté onion and garlic, add sweet potatoes and broth, and simmer until tender.

• Purée and stir in coconut milk.

Vegan Black Bean Soup

Ingredients:

• Black beans (canned)

• Bell peppers, onion, and garlic (chopped)

• Vegetable broth (low-sodium)

• Cumin and chili powder (ground)

Instructions:

• Sauté bell peppers, onion, and garlic until soft.

• Add beans, broth, and spices, and simmer.

• Purée half the soup for a thicker texture.

Vegan Gazpacho

Ingredients:

• Tomatoes, cucumbers, and bell peppers
(chopped)

• Red onion (finely chopped)

• Garlic (minced)

• Red wine vinegar and olive oil (low-sodium)

Instructions:

• Combine chopped vegetables, onion, and garlic.

• Add red wine vinegar and olive oil, then blend
until smooth.

Vegan Zucchini Soup

Ingredients:

• Zucchini (sliced)

• Onion and garlic (chopped)

• Vegetable broth (low-sodium)

• Fresh basil (chopped)

Instructions:

• Sauté onion and garlic, add zucchini and broth, and simmer until zucchini is tender.

• Purée and stir in fresh basil.

Vegan Red Lentil Soup

Ingredients:

• Red lentils

• Carrots, celery, and onions (chopped)

• Vegetable broth (low-sodium)

• Curry powder (for flavor)

Instructions:

• Sauté vegetables, add lentils, broth, and curry powder.

• Simmer until lentils are soft.

Vegan Cabbage Soup

Ingredients:

• Green cabbage (shredded)

• Carrots and onions (chopped)

• Vegetable broth (low-sodium)

• Smoked paprika (for flavor)

Instructions:

• Sauté carrots and onions, add cabbage and broth, and simmer until cabbage is tender.

• Season with smoked paprika.

Vegan Corn Chowder

Ingredients:

• Corn kernels (fresh or frozen)

• Potatoes (peeled and diced)

• Onion and garlic (chopped)

• Vegetable broth (low-sodium)

Instructions:

• Sauté onion and garlic, add corn, potatoes, and broth, and simmer until potatoes are soft.

Vegan Thai Tom Yum Soup

Ingredients:

• Mushrooms and tofu (sliced)

• Lemongrass, galangal (or ginger), and lime leaves (for flavor)

• Vegetable broth (low-sodium)

• Coconut milk (low-sodium)

Instructions:

• Sauté mushrooms and tofu, add lemongrass, galangal (or ginger), lime leaves, broth, and coconut milk.

• Simmer until flavors meld, then remove the aromatic ingredients.

DESSERTS

Vegan Chocolate Avocado Mousse

Ingredients:

• Ripe avocados

• Unsweetened cocoa powder

• Maple syrup (or other sweetener)

• Vanilla extract

Instructions:

• Blend avocados, cocoa powder, maple syrup, and vanilla extract until smooth and creamy.

• Chill before serving.

Vegan Banana Ice Cream

Ingredients:

• Ripe bananas (frozen)

Instructions:

• Blend frozen bananas until smooth.

• Customize with toppings like berries, nuts, or a drizzle of low-sodium chocolate sauce.

Vegan Date and Nut Bars

Ingredients:

• Dates

• Nuts (e.g., almonds, cashews)

• Unsweetened shredded coconut

Instructions:

• Blend dates and nuts in a food processor until they form a sticky mixture.

• Press into a pan, sprinkle with shredded coconut, and refrigerate until firm.

Vegan Chia Pudding

Ingredients:

• Chia seeds

• Unsweetened plant-based milk

• Vanilla extract

• Maple syrup (or other sweetener)

Instructions:

• Mix chia seeds, plant-based milk, vanilla extract, and maple syrup.

• Refrigerate until it thickens, then top with fresh fruit.

Vegan Oatmeal Cookies

Ingredients:

• Rolled oats

• Ripe bananas

• Unsweetened applesauce

• Cinnamon and vanilla extract

Instructions:

• Mash bananas and mix with oats, applesauce, cinnamon, and vanilla.

• Drop spoonfuls onto a baking sheet and bake until lightly browned.

Vegan Berry Crisp

Ingredients:

• Mixed berries (fresh or frozen)

• Rolled oats

• Almond meal

• Maple syrup (or other sweetener)

Instructions:

• Mix berries with a touch of maple syrup and spread in a baking dish.

• Combine rolled oats, almond meal, and a bit more maple syrup as the topping.

• Bake until the topping is golden and the berries are bubbly.

Vegan Rice Pudding

Ingredients:

• Arborio rice

- Coconut milk (low-sodium)

- Maple syrup (or other sweetener)

- Cinnamon and vanilla extract

Instructions:

- Cook rice in coconut milk with maple syrup, cinnamon, and vanilla until creamy.

- Serve warm or chilled.

Vegan Chocolate Chip Cookies

Ingredients:

- Whole wheat flour

- Unsweetened applesauce

- Chocolate chips (low-sodium)

- Baking powder

Instructions:

• Mix flour, applesauce, chocolate chips, and baking powder to form a dough.

• Drop spoonfuls onto a baking sheet and bake until golden.

Vegan Fruit Salad

Ingredients:

• Assorted fresh fruit (e.g., berries, melon, citrus)

• Fresh mint (chopped)

• Lime juice (optional)

Instructions:

• Toss fresh fruit with chopped mint and a squeeze of lime juice if desired.

Vegan Chocolate-Dipped Strawberries

Ingredients:

• Fresh strawberries

• Vegan chocolate chips (low-sodium)

Instructions:

• Melt vegan chocolate chips in the microwave or on a stovetop.

• Dip strawberries in the melted chocolate and let them cool on parchment paper.

Vegan Blueberry Muffins

Ingredients:

• Whole wheat flour

• Blueberries (fresh or frozen)

• Unsweetened applesauce

• Baking powder and cinnamon

Instructions:

• Mix flour, blueberries, applesauce, baking powder, and cinnamon.

• Fill muffin cups and bake until golden.

Vegan Coconut Rice Pudding

Ingredients:

• Arborio rice

• Coconut milk (low-sodium)

• Agave syrup (or other sweetener)

• Shredded coconut (unsweetened)

Instructions:

• Cook rice in coconut milk with agave syrup until creamy.

• Stir in shredded coconut and serve.

Vegan Apple Crisp

Ingredients:

• Apples (sliced)

• Rolled oats

• Almond meal

• Cinnamon and nutmeg

Instructions:

• Mix sliced apples with a sprinkle of cinnamon and nutmeg, and place in a baking dish.

• Combine rolled oats and almond meal as the crisp topping.

• Bake until the apples are tender and the topping is golden.

Vegan Lemon Sorbet

Ingredients:

• Lemon juice (freshly squeezed)

• Agave syrup (or other sweetener)

Instructions:

• Mix lemon juice and agave syrup.

• Freeze in an ice cream maker or a shallow container, stirring occasionally until firm.

Vegan Pomegranate and Orange Parfait

Ingredients:

• Pomegranate seeds

• Orange segments

• Coconut yogurt (unsweetened)

• Chopped nuts (e.g., almonds or walnuts)

Instructions:

• Layer pomegranate seeds, orange segments, and coconut yogurt in a glass.

• Top with chopped nuts.

Vegan Hummus and Veggie Sticks

Ingredients:

• Chickpeas (canned)

• Tahini

• Lemon juice

• Garlic (minced)

• Carrot, cucumber, and bell pepper sticks

Instructions:

• Blend chickpeas, tahini, lemon juice, and minced garlic to make hummus.

• Serve with fresh veggie sticks for dipping.

Vegan Guacamole and Whole Wheat Pita Triangles

Ingredients:

- Ripe avocados

- Tomato (diced)

- Onion (finely chopped)

- Lime juice

- Whole wheat pita bread (cut into triangles)

Instructions:

- Mash avocados and mix with diced tomato, chopped onion, and lime juice.

- Serve with whole wheat pita triangles.

Vegan Trail Mix

Ingredients:

- Mixed nuts (unsalted)

- Dried fruits (e.g., raisins, apricots)

- Dark chocolate chips (low-sodium)

- Pumpkin seeds

Instructions:

• Combine mixed nuts, dried fruits, dark chocolate chips, and pumpkin seeds in a bowl.

• Portion into snack-sized bags for easy grab-and-go.

Vegan Rice Cakes with Nut Butter and Banana Slices

Ingredients:

• Rice cakes (low-sodium)

• Nut butter (e.g., almond or peanut)

• Ripe banana (sliced)

Instructions:

• Spread nut butter on rice cakes and top with banana slices.

Vegan Edamame

Ingredients:

• Edamame beans (frozen)

• Sea salt (optional)

Instructions:

• Steam edamame beans until tender.

• Sprinkle with a pinch of sea salt if desired.

Vegan Baked Sweet Potato Fries

Ingredients:

• Sweet potatoes (cut into fries)

• Olive oil (low-sodium)

• Paprika and garlic powder

Instructions:

• Toss sweet potato fries with olive oil, paprika, and garlic powder.

• Bake until crispy.

Vegan Popcorn

Ingredients:

• Popcorn kernels

• Nutritional yeast (for flavor)

• Olive oil (low-sodium)

Instructions:

• Air-pop popcorn or pop it with a small amount of olive oil.

• Sprinkle with nutritional yeast for a cheesy flavor.

Vegan Sliced Apples with Almond Butter

Ingredients:

• Apples (sliced)

• Almond butter (unsalted)

Instructions:

• Spread almond butter on apple slices for a tasty
and nutritious snack.

Vegan Cucumber Slices with Hummus

Ingredients:

• Cucumber (sliced)

• Hummus

Instructions:

• Use cucumber slices as dippers for hummus.

Vegan Roasted Chickpeas

Ingredients:

• Chickpeas (canned, drained, and rinsed)

• Olive oil (low-sodium)

• Spices (e.g., paprika, cumin, chili powder)

Instructions:

• Toss chickpeas with olive oil and spices.

• Roast in the oven until crispy.

Vegan Greek Yogurt with Berries

Ingredients:

• Plant-based Greek yogurt (unsweetened)

• Mixed berries (fresh or frozen)

• Agave syrup (or other sweetener)

Instructions:

• Top plant-based Greek yogurt with mixed berries and a drizzle of agave syrup.

Vegan Energy Balls

Ingredients:

• Dates

• Rolled oats

- Almonds

- Nut butter

- Cocoa powder (unsweetened)

Instructions:

- Blend dates, rolled oats, almonds, nut butter, and cocoa powder in a food processor.

- Form into balls and refrigerate.

Vegan Salsa and Baked Tortilla Chips

Ingredients:

- Whole wheat tortillas (cut into triangles)

- Low-sodium salsa

Instructions:

- Bake tortilla triangles until crispy.

- Serve with low-sodium salsa.

Vegan Veggie Roll-Ups

Ingredients:

• Large lettuce leaves (e.g., Romaine or iceberg)

• Hummus

• Sliced veggies (e.g., bell peppers, carrots)

Instructions:

• Spread hummus on lettuce leaves and add sliced veggies.

• Roll up and enjoy!

Vegan Fruit Kabobs

Ingredients:

• Assorted fruits (e.g., pineapple, melon, berries)

• Wooden skewers

Instructions:

• Thread chunks of assorted fruits onto wooden skewers for a colorful and refreshing snack.

A low-sodium plant-based cookbook offers a valuable resource for individuals looking to embrace a healthier, plant-centric lifestyle while managing their sodium intake. This type of cookbook provides a wealth of delicious and nutritious recipes that prioritize whole, unprocessed plant foods while minimizing sodium content.

The cookbook includes a variety of recipes, spanning from appetizers and main dishes to desserts and snacks. These recipes are designed to meet the dietary needs of those aiming to reduce their sodium intake, whether it's for health reasons or simply to promote overall well-being.

By using creative and flavorful alternatives to salt, such as herbs, spices, and other seasonings, these cookbooks empower individuals to enjoy a wide range of satisfying meals without compromising taste. Additionally, the inclusion of nutrient-dense ingredients like vegetables, fruits, whole grains, legumes, and nuts ensures that these recipes are not only low in sodium but also packed with essential vitamins, minerals, and fiber.

Overall, a low-sodium plant-based cookbook serves as a valuable tool for those seeking to improve their health, lower their blood pressure, or simply explore the delicious world of plant-based cuisine. It encourages individuals to make informed dietary choices and embrace a lifestyle that is both heart-healthy and environmentally conscious. Whether you're a seasoned plant-based eater or new to the concept, this cookbook can inspire and guide you on a path toward better health and well-being.